Practical Experienced Method for
Natural Pain Relief

TURN PAIN OFF

A Self-Help Guide to Alleviate Musculoskeletal Pain Using Trigger Point Relief Technique

L. HEHIR

MScAc, RGN, SCM, EFT Ad-cert

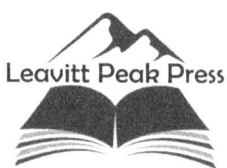

ISBN: 978-1-969865-64-0 (sc)
ISBN: 978-1-969865-65-7 (e)

Rev. date: 12/09/2025

This book being a slightly newer version has a bit more detail than the audio version.

CONTENTS

OVERVIEW

As a qualified Traditional Chinese Medicine Acupuncturist and a retired nurse after serving the NHS for 41 years I decided to write this book with the aim to provide support and guidance to all people who may be suffering from musculo-skeletal pain (the muscles attached to the skeletal frame to support it). This book contains predominantly information from the perspective of Traditional Chinese Medicine with linkages being made to western Medicine. It is designed to be used as a supplement to western Medicine and not to replace it.

This simplified easy to use self-help guide provides you with information on how to use acupressure to release trigger points in your shoulders, upper and lower back and limbs only that are possibly giving rise to your musculoskeletal pain. **It should be noted that acupressure to the neck area should not be undertaken at home.** Illustrated stretches for the neck area are depicted and may be used.

It is highly recommended that you consult a doctor prior to considering any form of self-treatment to ensure it is safe to do so.

The guide has been designed to help you gain relief from pain and improve mobility. Although it primarily focuses on the upper body, the principles can be applied to pain on lower back, buttocks and limbs to allow you to gain relief from musculoskeletal pain.

The guide describes what trigger points are, how trigger points develop, how they cause pain and suggests an acupressure trigger point technique to release the trigger points. It illustrates where you may be feeling the pain, where the common trigger points can be found and muscles stretches that can be undertaken following release of the trigger point in order to prevent them reoccurring.

The technique is **not applicable for the neck, directly on the spine, abdomen or frontal chest area.** Seek medical advice and professional practitioner support for treating trigger points in these areas.

CAUTION

Neither should it be used for more complex painful chronic conditions e.g.

- **Fibromyalgia or**
- **Complex Regional Pain Syndrome (CRPS),**
- **Neuritis, neuropathy or other nerve or spinal conditions.**
- **Rheumatoid Arthritis**
- **Other Medical conditions e.g. Lupus, Shingles etc.**

Or

- **On an area of skin that is broken or infected**
- **Or directly over bruised skin (for bruises work above or below)**

If you have a cold or flu or any other form of general illness.

NOTE: **More complex chronic conditions** are best treated by professionals e.g. local pain control doctors, physiotherapists and or Traditional Chinese Medicine acupuncturists among others. (See British Acupuncture Council for qualified acupuncturists in your area or similar Regulatory councils in your individual countries.)

INTRODUCTION

During the natural course of our daily activities we can put a great deal of stress on our bodies. Much of this stress can affect the flexibility and function of our skeletal muscles, whether it is from sports, bad posture, work activities, over-stretching, repetitive actions or emotional and psychologically traumatizing events in our lives. Osteoarthritis (wear and tear of joint(s) can also put stress on our muscles. The joint(s) can become distorted pulling on the tendons and muscles and lead to over stretching causing pain.

The effect on the muscles from these stressors can diminish the free flow of energy and blood in our muscles and or cause areas where the flow becomes constricted from muscles becoming too tight and contracted and a trigger point arises causing pain and or stiffness.

The skeletal muscles within our bodies can be prone to developing areas of localised constriction (trigger point) from tense/tight muscles. Sometimes the pain can be felt at a distance from where the actual constriction is. Pain at a distance from the trigger point is known as referred pain, whereas pain at the trigger point site is described as localised pain.

Using a trigger point relief technique on the affected muscle or muscles can help the muscles to relax and lead to an alleviation of the blockage and pain being felt. The technique described in this book is based on acupressure both on acupuncture points and painful, tight muscle points elsewhere. It is possible to apply acupressure on yourself in the comfort of your own home. Acupressure is suitable for localised and referred pain and is worth trying for muscle pain.

FORMATION OF MUSCLE TRIGGER POINTS

The muscles throughout our body that are attached to our bones are known as skeletal muscles. Skeletal muscles are composed of bundles of muscle fibres or bands that have the ability to contract (shorten) and relax (lengthen) to produce body movement and can be activated voluntarily by our thoughts to move e.g. when we want to walk etc.

Messages sent via the nervous system to nerves in the muscles stimulate movement by causing a number of muscles to contract and relax at different times. The stressors' previously mentioned, can result in one or more muscle bands or part of a band to fail to relax properly. When a part of a band does not relax fully the whole of the band is being held tense and can feel like a tight guitar string when felt under the skin. The part of the muscle band that fails to relax completely can feel like a hard knot deep within the muscle, be extremely sensitive to touch or pressure and can characteristically cause pain elsewhere in the body. This is what is known as a trigger point. Depending on the stressors more than one trigger point may have developed. Also if one muscle is failing to relax this can impact on other adjoining muscles giving rise to more than one trigger point.

For example: emotional and psychological stress usually affects the muscles in the shoulder and upper back. When we feel stressed or under pressure we tend to hold our shoulders, back and sometimes neck tense. When these muscles are held tight for lengthy periods their ability to relax may be diminished over time. This can give rise to a number of trigger points. Although some stress is good constantly feeling stressed could possibly continuously give rise to trigger points so it is important to take steps to deal with the stress.

Common Back Trigger Points

Figure 1 illustrates the possible areas where common trigger points can be found. The model also depicts that many trigger points can be found on or close to acupuncture points.

Figure 1: Upper Back Trigger Point Sites

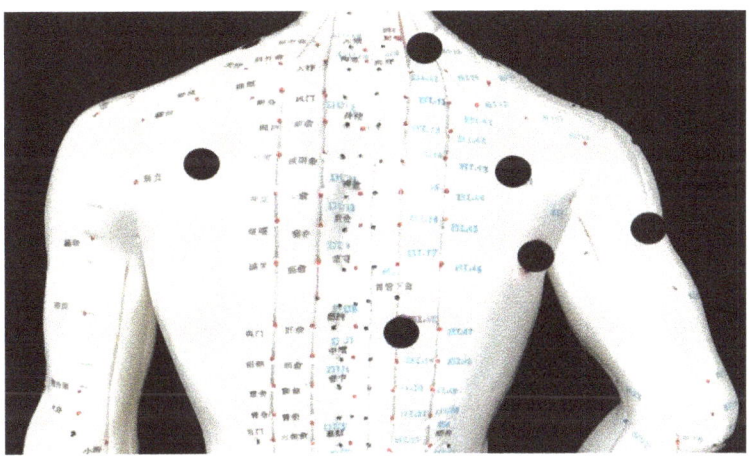

D.G Travell and J Simons in their book Myofascial Pain and Dysfunction Volume 1 and 2 for acupuncture practitioners identifies common sites throughout the body where trigger points can occur as depicted on the models as black dots in *Figures 1 and 2a and b.*

Figure 2a & b: Common Lower Body Trigger Point Sites

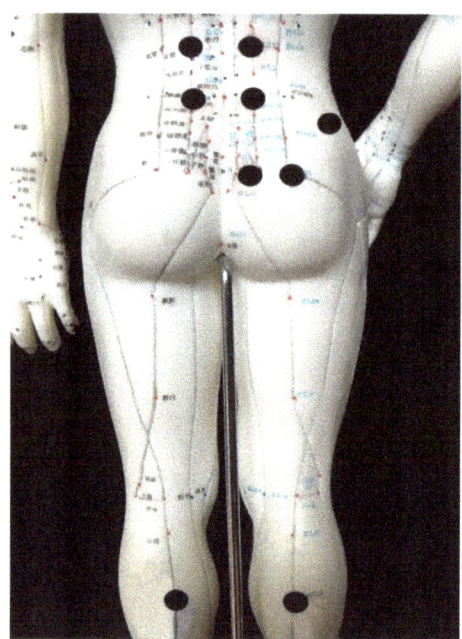
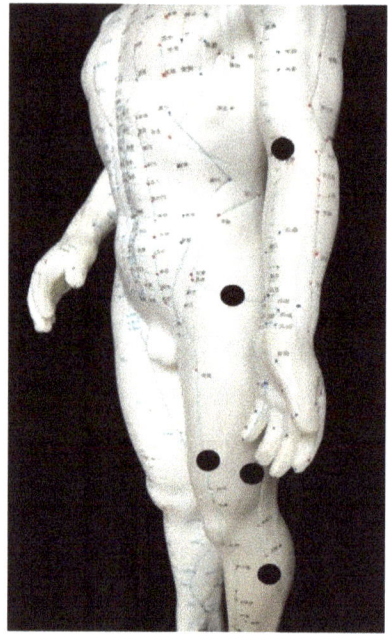

Pain results when the muscle stays in a contracted or shortened state, (instead of relaxing), from the constant pressure being applied on the nerves because they are being held too tightly by the muscle. The pressure can be directly on nerve endings (as identified by Travell and Simons), which causes severe pain at the site of the trigger point. Whereas, pain felt in other parts of the body distant from the trigger point can be related to the muscle contraction trapping nerves that pass through the muscle to other parts of the body.

The contraction of the muscle also compresses the blood vessels passing through the muscles and may cause an obstruction to the free flow of the blood in and out of this area, which increases the pain. Arterial blood carries oxygen and nutrient materials required to keep the muscles healthy and if a muscle does not receive these nutrients it can become weakened. Also, when muscles contract chemical waste materials are produced and when in a relaxed state the waste materials are carried away by the blood for excretion from the body.

If waste products are not fully removed, the muscle may become more irritated, the contraction will continue and more pain will result. The contracted muscle can also be irritated further by being overstimulated in the case of long constant deep pressure or too much rubbing and kneading.

ACUPRESSURE AND TRIGGER POINTS

Acupressure is part of ancient Traditional Chinese Medicine treatments and is commonly used on trigger points or painful points. Qualified acupuncturists can either needle and or use acupressure on these points to help with many types of conditions of the body. Acupressure is about applying pressure or vibrational movements. For the purposes of self treatment the acupressure technique described is about applying slow gentle to progressively deeper pressure on the trigger point.

The aim is to alleviate the pain by relaxing the muscles without causing added pain if possible, and by promoting the free flow of blood for providing the nutrients for feeding the muscle and removal of the waste materials and to allow the muscles to return to their normal length and function. Using acupressure on the trigger points can help with relaxing the affected muscle and promote the free flow of blood and energy.

Pressure on the contracted muscle or trigger point can cause pain elsewhere in the body, this is known as 'pain referral'. However even when pressure only causes pain at the site where the pressure is being applied and a muscular knot is or not felt, it is still worth using the acupressure technique to relax the muscle.

When nerves passing through the muscles become trapped at a trigger point site, pain may be felt in other parts of the body and not at the trigger point site itself. This is known as 'referred pain'. For example, trigger points in the shoulder, neck or chest, which may or may not be painful on touch, can cause you to feel pain in your arm.

Although finding the trigger point(s) can be tricky and requires patience, the following information has been provided as a guide to illustrate where to search and the technique to use.

The yellow shading on the models arm in *Figure 3* illustrates where pain may be being felt on the body. Whilst the black dots illustrate where trigger points may be found.

Figure 3: Referred Pain Site and Trigger points.

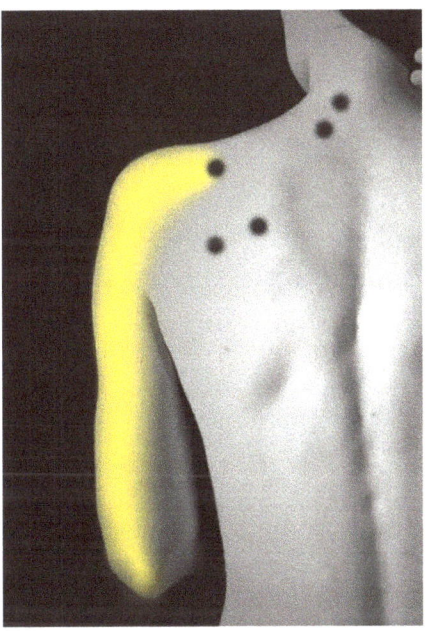

Referred pain from trigger points can be felt, as headaches or migraines, joint or muscle pain, pain and stiffness in the back or elsewhere and shooting type pain down the legs (sciatica type pain) or arms. Trigger points constricting nerves in the muscle may also give rise to burning sensations, pins and needles or numbness and tingling.

More complex painful muscle conditions such as **Fibromyalgia** or **Complex Regional Pain Syndrome** (CRPS), **Neuritis or other nerve conditions** are best treated by professionals e.g. local pain control doctors, physiotherapists and or Traditional Chinese Medicine acupuncturists among others. (See British Acupuncture Council for qualified acupuncturists in your area or similar Councils in your individual countries.

SEARCHING FOR KNOTS OR TRIGGER POINTS IN THE MUSCLES

When feeling for painful spots or knots in the muscles use either the soft padded distal end of thumb, fingers or knuckles or ask a partner, friend, or family member to do so if the pain is in an area that you cannot reach.

- Start by feeling around the area where the pain is for sensitive areas and or hard muscle knots. Do this gently but use sufficient pressure to allow you to feel any hard knots or tightness deep in the muscle.
- If pain is felt on a limb work upwards moving towards the main body. For example if you are having pain in an arm move up to feel around your shoulder and back area close to the shoulder, for painful knots as well as in the arm itself. If pain is felt in leg, feel around your buttock area, either side of the lower spine area as well as along the track of the pain in the leg. See **Figures 2a, b and c** above for suggested areas to search for common trigger points. Other images are depicted below showing more specific points.
- Remember there can be more than one trigger point. So even after you have dealt with one trigger point feel around further to make sure there are no others, but do this in stages and not all at the same time. If you cannot find a knot but feel a tight muscle band it is still worth using the technique on the band.
- Even if there is a painful spot that feels knotted but is not causing further pain when pressure is applied or causing pain elsewhere; it is still worth dealing with. This will help towards avoiding future referred pain and a chronic pain.

ACUPRESSURE RELIEF TECHNIQUE FOR TRIGGER POINTS

ACUPRESSURE IS NOT TO BE USED ON THE NECK OR DIRECTLY ON THE SPINE .

STRETCHES HAVE BEEN PROVIDED FOR NECK TRIGGER POINTS.

This acupressure technique for trigger point to help relax your muscle(s) is to be applied directly onto the trigger point itself if found, but is also worth doing on tight muscles. I have personally found that pushing inwards at a slight angle on the knot or tightness in the muscle (as if you were pushing it deeper and slightly away from where it lies in the body) can be more successful than applying pressure by pushing directly inwards only. Only use the technique for a maximum of 2 minutes at any given time.

Preparing for the technique

Warming your muscles by showering/ bathing or holding a warming device (e.g. hot water bottle wrapped in towel to avoid burns) to the area can help soften the muscle, before undertaking the following technique. A thin layer of clothing can be worn.

BEFORE TREATING

- Drink a glass of water before and after using the technique.
- Before beginning take 3 deep breaths to help your general relaxation.

- Make yourself comfortable and in a position where you can reach the parts of the body you need to reach.

Note on Pressure

- For best result and to avoid unnecessary pain, apply the pressure gently then increase the pressure slowly but firmly using the soft padded end of a thumb or finger (whichever feels most comfortable for you). Or if you are working on the buttocks I find using a knuckle works best.

The Acupressure Technique

- 10 second treatment. Apply slight pressure on the knot or tight muscle, take a deep breath and hold your breath for 2 - 4 seconds, then release the breath slowly. Start applying more pressure when holding your breath and continue to increase the pressure gently on the trigger point/ tight muscle/ muscle knot as you release your breath slowly. When pain is felt ease off the pressure slightly until pain is no longer felt and continue to hold until the 10 seconds is up.
- After the 10 seconds are up, release all pressure for 5 seconds then repeat the pressure technique again, once more on the same area. It is then good to adjust where you are applying the pressure to slightly above and/or below where the knot is felt to avoid overstimulating the knot and to encourage more movement/relaxation of the knot.
- Keep doing this with slight adjustments on the muscle position until no pain is felt with deep pressure and the knot in the muscle has softened or for a **maximum time of 2 minutes.**
- If there has been no change in the intensity of the pain felt during the 2 minutes, this may suggest either that the muscle has not softened or the pressure is being applied to a nerve ending. If

it has not softened it will require repeat treatments up to two to three times in a day. However you can change the position of where you apply the pressure to further above or below the knotted area.

- If the pain felt on pressure is too strong this suggests it is over a nerve ending. Therefore apply the pressure to above and below the trigger point.
- Also you may find that even though the pain did not decrease at the time of applying the pressure that the pain eases off as you go about your day.
- After applying pressure and releasing the trigger point(s), the relaxed muscle should be stretched. If the muscles are not returned to normal length, there is a greater likelihood the Trigger Points will reoccur. Stretching can be less painful after the trigger points has been reduced. Stretch the muscle when it has relaxed by using two fingers or both hand on either side of where the knot was/is. Then move the limbs or head etc. to stretch the muscles further using the stretch images on the following pages for guidance.
- It can also be helpful to say positive affirmations to yourself during this process e.g. I acknowledge this pain and now allow my muscles to relax, I am grateful that my muscles are functioning normally or I let go any stress that may be contributing to this pain.
- Saying affirmation instructs your brain to release the pain. For further information check out Emotional Freedom Techniques.
- *TIP:* If you don't have anyone to help with the pain in your back, place a tennis ball inside a long sock or stocking – place it on the floor and lie on it. Adjust the tennis ball using the extra length of the sock until it is directly under where the trigger point/knot is. Roll off the ball every 5-10 seconds, keep doing this for about 2 minutes maximum until pain is reduced, then do the muscle stretches.

MUSCLE PAIN SITES AND TRIGGER POINT IMAGES

The following section uses images to depict the sites where pain may be being felt, where trigger points may be located and suggested movements for stretching the muscle, to help release the trigger points and prevent further reoccurrence.

The shaded yellow areas on the images below indicate where you may be feeling pain and the black dots or crosses identify possible sites where trigger points can be found. The referred pain will occur on the same side of the body as the trigger points. This is a general guide only to help you source your Trigger Points.

HEAD, NECK, SHOULDER AND UPPER BACK PAIN

The yellow shaded areas illustrate the referred pain areas associated with trigger points in the trapezius upper back muscle can be felt in a variety of different areas as illustrated by the yellow areas in *Figure 4 a, b, c. & d.*

Figure 4a, b, c &d: Head, Neck, Shoulder or Upper Back

Possible Referred Pain Sites.

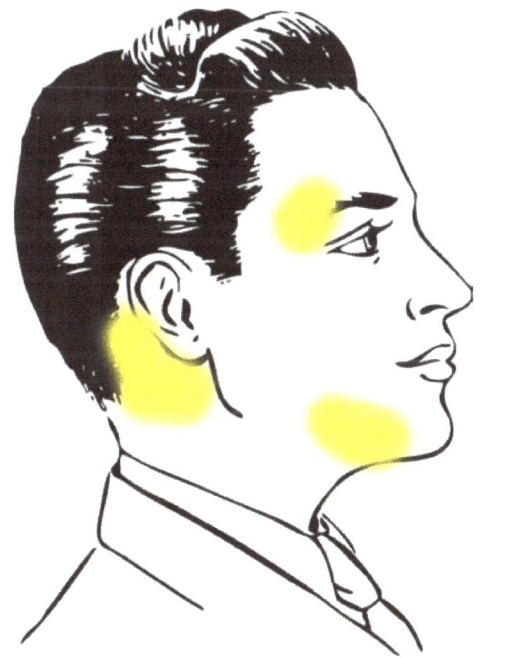
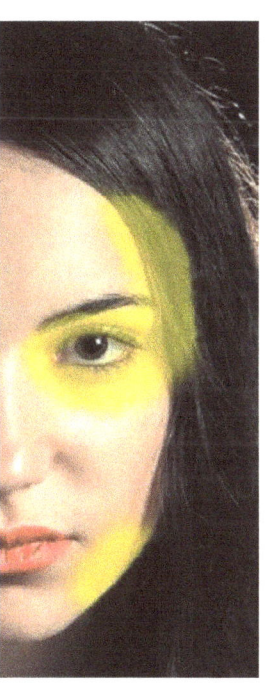

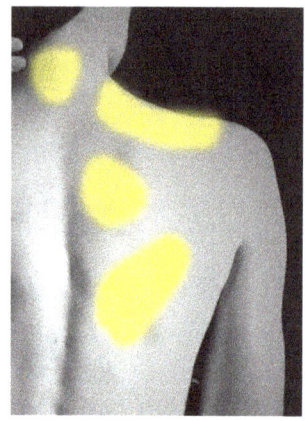
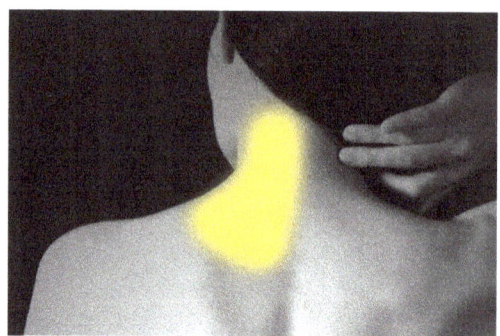

The black dots in *Figure 5* illustrate locations where trigger points may be found which could be causing referred pain shown in *Figures 4 a, b, c or d.*

Figure 5: Head, Neck Shoulder and Upper Back Pain Trigger Points

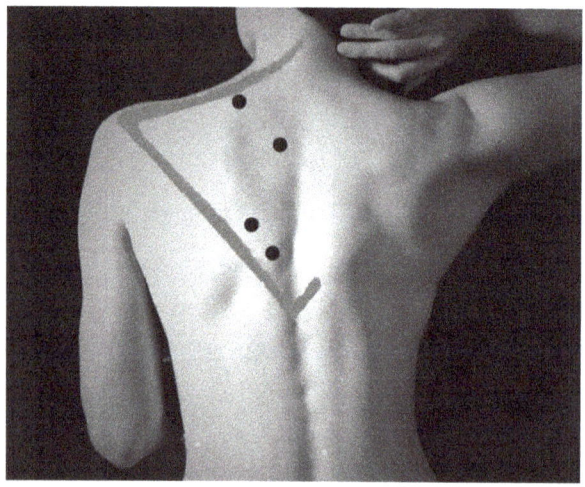

The neck has major vessels and nerves within it, so it is highly recommended that you do not attempt to release trigger points on the the neck itself and seek medical / dentist professional advice as required.

Figure 6 & 9: Shows stretch exercise as the recommended treatment for the neck trigger points.

Figure 6: Upper Back and Side Neck Stretch With Explanation.

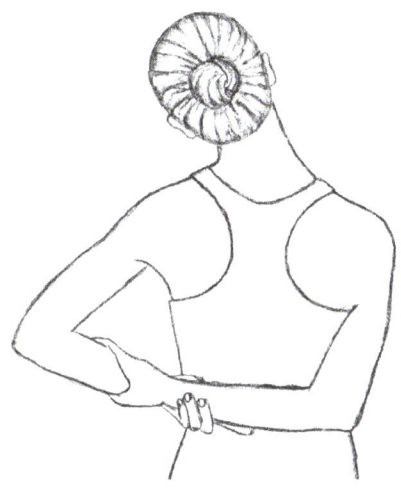

Place right arm behind back, and grasp wrist with left hand, as shown.

Bend neck sideways to the left while pulling on right arm.

Hold for 10-15 seconds, release and repeat twice more.

Repeat for other side. Undertake at least three times daily.

The yellow shaded are in *Figure 7* illustrates the pain location when there are trigger points in the Levator Scapulae Muscles at the back of the neck. *Figure 8* illustrates where you may find two common trigger points for the pain felt.

Figure 7: Neck Pain Area

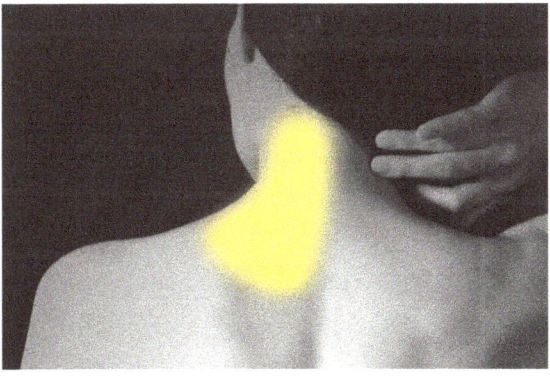

Figure 8 Trigger Point Locations

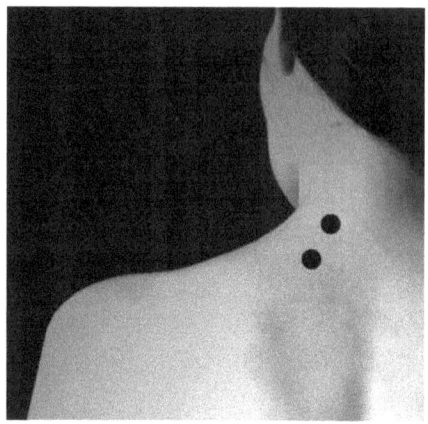

Figure 9: Back & Side of the Neck Stretch

Sit on chair. Grasp seat of chair with right hand.

Stretch the Levator scapula muscles by placing left hand on head and gently pull over to the side and slightly forward.

Hold for 10-15 seconds, repeat three times.

Repeat for other side.

Do this at least three times daily.

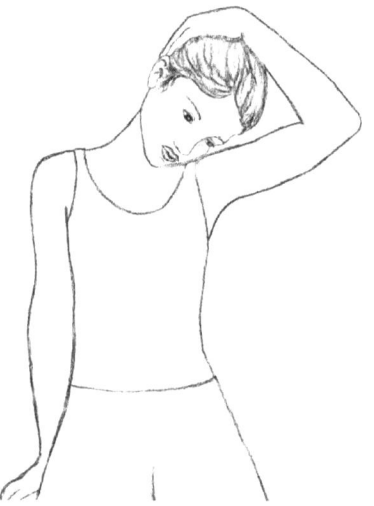

The back of the neck muscles also include the Capitis and Trapezium muscles. Headaches like a tight band round the head or migraines are commonly associated with trigger points in the muscles at back of the neck. Remember do not attempt to release these trigger points, however the stretch exercises can be undertaken.

Figure 11 illustrates where trigger points may be found for headaches felt like a tight band around the head (**Figure 10**) and or dull pain at the top of the head.

Figure 10: Referred Pain Sites

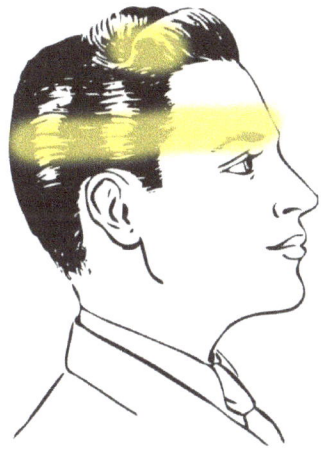

Figure 11 Trigger Points Site

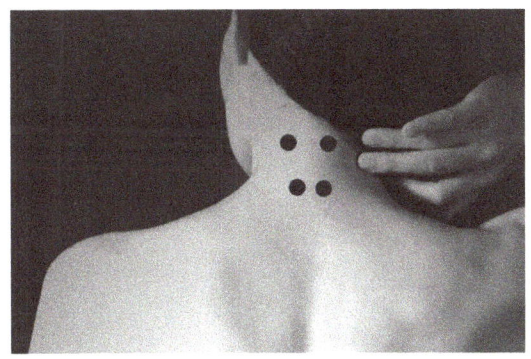

Figure 12: Back of Neck Stretch

Place hand on back of head.

Gently encourage chin towards chest.

Avoid any force.

Hold for 10-15 seconds; repeat three times

Undertake at least three times daily.

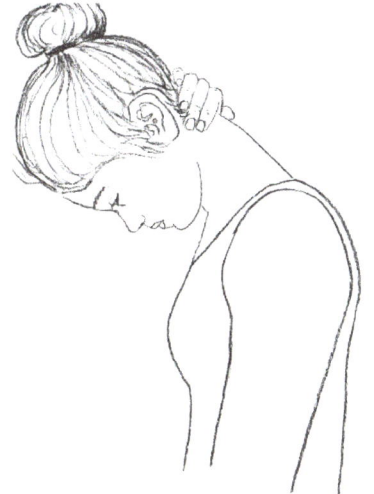

Front and Side of Neck Trigger Points & Referred Pain.

Trigger points in the front of neck or the side of the neck can give rise to front of the head headaches as well as facial pain, teeth and tongue pain.

They can also cause balance or hearing problems due to disturbances in the inner ear and eye problems e.g drooping lid, red and or weeping eyes.

The following stretch may be beneficial in releasing a trigger point without the need for pressure being applied.

Figure 13: Front of Neck Stretch

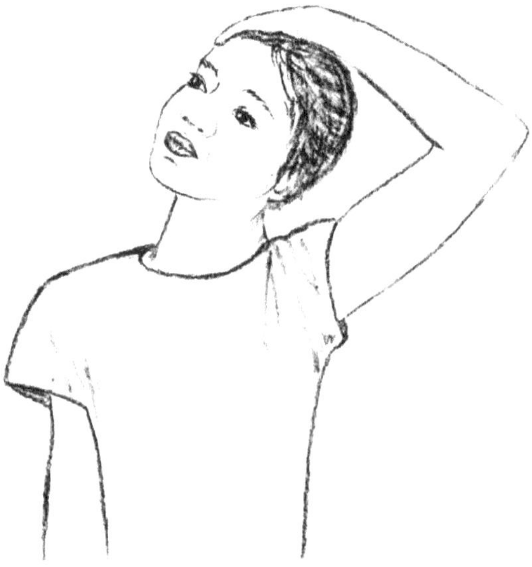

Sit on chair. Grasp seat of chair with right hand.

To stretch the Sternocleidomastoid muscle place left hand on head and gently pull head toward the left shoulder.

Maintain light pressure and turn head to the right.

Hold for 10-15 seconds. Repeat three times.

Repeat for other side of the neck. Undertake at least three times daily.

Figure 15: Side and Front of the Neck Stretch

HOLD left wrist behind back. Lower left shoulder, and then tilt your head to the right.

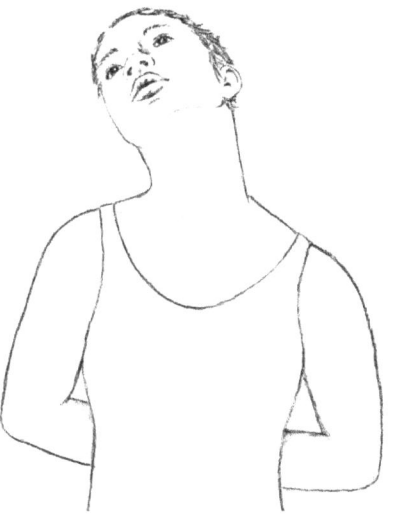

Slowly roll head backwards until a stretch is felt.

Hold for 10-15 seconds.

Undertake three times.

Repeat for other side. Repeat three times daily.

CHEST, ARM AND BACK PAIN

The pressure technique is not to for use on the front aspect of the chest.

This part is for information only.

The yellow shaded areas in Figure 14a & b illustrate where referred pain may be felt from trigger points in the scalene muscles in the side of the neck.

Figure 14a & b: Scalene Muscles Referred Pain

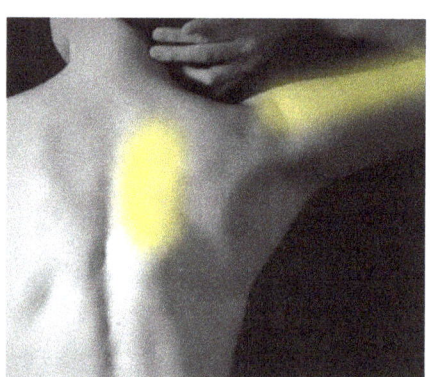 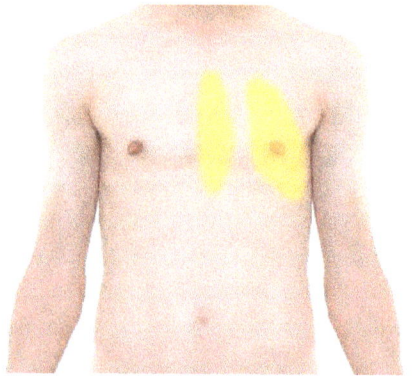

Pain in these muscles and may be related to more than trigger points and cause a number of symptoms.

Always seek medical advice for the following symptoms.

Symptoms may include chest angina type pain, numbness, tingling, swelling and weakness of the arms and hands. It is highly recommended that a professional carry out treatment if appropriate depending on the cause.

See next page for back trigger points.

UPPER BACK PAIN

Figure 16 illustrates where back pain may be felt and the possible location of the trigger points, when the deep Rhomboid back muscles are involved. Trigger points in the Rhomboid muscles are extremely painful and can be chronic in nature. Acupressure technique can be used here.

Figure 16: Rhomboid Muscle – Pain Area and Trigger Points

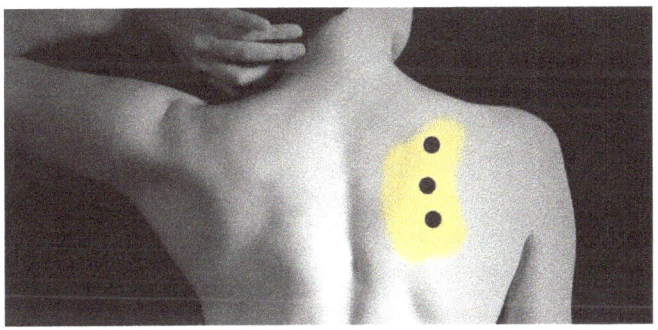

Figure 17: Rhomboid Stretch

Bring left arm across front of body as shown.

Stretch the muscle by holding elbow with right arm and gently pull arm across chest.

Hold for 10-15 seconds.

Do this three times.

Repeat for other side.

Repeat at least three times a day.

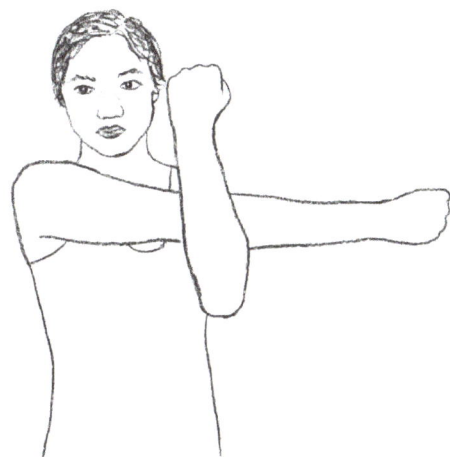

Figure 18 illustrates where back pain may be felt and the possible location of the trigger points, when the muscles that run parallel with the spine (e.g. the Erector Spinae or Semi Spinalis Capitis muscles) are involved. **Seek professional help.**

Tense/stiff muscles on either side of the spine can pull it out of alignment, resulting in a chronic deformity of the spine. There may also be abdominal pain associated with nerves being trapped exiting the spine.

Figure 18: Pain Areas and Trigger Point Locations

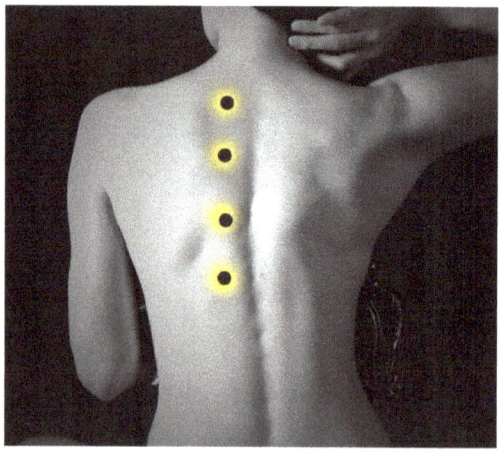

Figure 19: Parallel Spinal Muscles Stretch

Sit in slightly forward and firmly on chair.

To stretch the muscles cross arms at mid forearm, and slowly roll forward pushing your upper back up, until a stretch is felt.

Hold for 10-15 seconds.

Repeat three times.

Undertake at least three times a day.

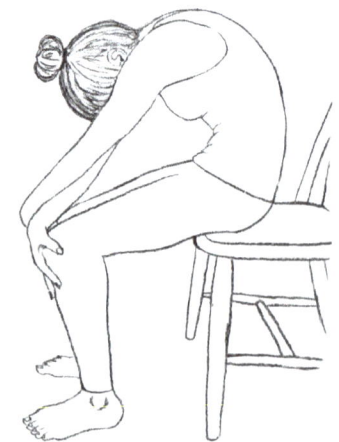

SCIATICA TYPE PAIN

Pain described as Sciatica may be caused by trigger points in the buttock muscles or muscles on either side of the spine - **see figure 2a**, therefore it is worth checking for any knotted areas in these muscles.

Figure 20 illustrates where pain may be felt in yellow and red (red area more severe) and the possible location of the trigger points.

Figure 20: Buttock muscles—Referred
Pain and Trigger Points Location

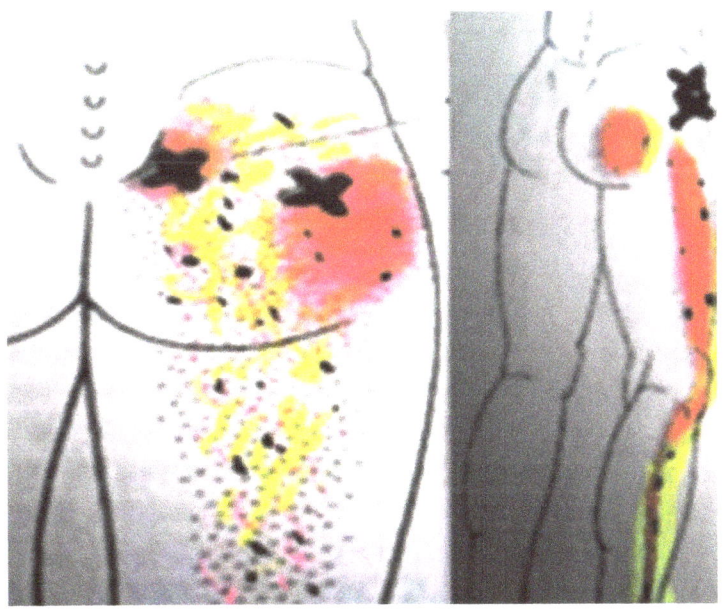

A number of stretching exercises for the buttock muscles may be used to help decrease the painful symptoms along the sciatic nerve and to improve motion function.

It is possible to use the acupressure technique on the points marked with a cross.

Sciatica Stretches

Figure 21a & b: Buttock Muscle Stretches.

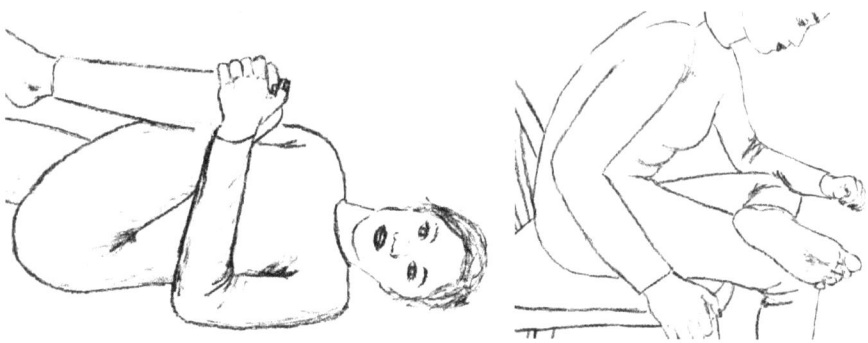

Figure 21a: Gluteal Stretch.	Figure 21b: Piriformis Muscle
Lie on a bed or floor. Using your hands bring your knee towards your opposite shoulder. Avoid over stretching.	**Stretch.** Sitting on a chair cross one leg over the other, resting your ankle on the opposite leg. Gently press down on the inside of the upper knee with your elbow and slowly lean forward until you feel a mild stretch.

For these stretches only go as far as you can without giving yourself added pain. Try to stretch the muscles further each time you do them.

Hold for 10 -15 seconds; repeat four times. Undertake at least twice a day.

SOME LIFESTYLE TIPS:

- Undertake muscle stretches each morning, before and after exercise or playing sport.
- Sleeping on a large pillow or more than one pillow may be distorting your neck and spine. Try reducing the height of your pillows. When sitting try as much as possible keep your neck and head in alignment with your spine.
- If working at a desk all day long, try and have your knees at a lower level than your hips; this will help your posture alignment. Stand and stretch every 20 minutes or so for a few minutes.
- If constantly working on a computer ensure your back is held straight and undertake hand and arm exercises every 20 minutes or so. For example: roll hand into a fist and release a number of times. Stretch arm high above your head hold and release. Stretch neck muscles as per above.
- Warm baths can help relax muscles.
- Avoid wallets being in back pockets, so that you are not sitting on them constantly.
- There is growing evidence of the benefits of meditation for deep relaxation. There are a number of free meditation videos online that can help guide you to meditate.
- Take action to reduce stress levels.

AUTHORS NOTE

I believe that no one should have to suffer from pain unnecessarily so I truly hope that you have found the information in this book understandable, useful and helpful in alleviating your pain. If you have not found any relief from your pain through the western medicine approach or from this material, I wish for you not to give up, but to try other complementary therapies (Acupuncture Practitioners, Chiropractors, Osteopaths, EFT practitioners, meditation and or therapeutic practitioners).

ACKNOWLEDGMENTS

I am grateful to Kate Copp and Anu Sharma, for proof reading this book and their suggestions. Also I thank Melanie Khodayar, for producing the stretch drawings.

REFERENCED MATERIAL

D.G. Travell and J Simons: Myofascial Pain and Dysfunction. The Trigger Point Manual. Volume 1 & 2. November 1998

D Finando & Stephen Finando, Trigger Point Therapy, for Myofascial Pain ; Healing Arts, August 2005.

www.ingramcontent.com/pod-product-compliance
Lightning Source LLC
Chambersburg PA
CBHW051252120626
46547CB00014B/1908